C000217290

BOOK 3

100 MCQs
ON
GASTROENTEROLOGY,
ENDOCRINOLOGY
AND
RENAL MEDICINE

Andrew D Higham MRCP
Training Fellow and Honorary Senior Registrar
Department of Gastroenterology
Hope Hospital, Salford

Colin M Dayan MA MRCP PhD
Consultant Senior Lecturer in Medicine
Bristol Royal Infirmary

Philip A Kalra MA MRCP MD
Consultant Nephrologist
Hope Hospital, Salford

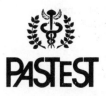

PASTEST

© 1997 PASTEST
Egerton Court, Parkgate Estate,
Knutsford, Cheshire, WA16 8DX

First edition 1987
Second edition 1997

A catalogue record for this book is available from the British Library.

ISBN: 0 906896 68 1

Typeset by Breeze Limited, Manchester
Printed by Bookmag, Inverness

CONTENTS

Introduction   v

MCQs on Gastroenterology   1

MCQs on Endocrinology   21

MCQs on Renal Medicine   45

Answers and teaching explanations are on the
back of each question page

Revision Checklist – Gastroenterology   67

Revision Checklist – Endocrinology   68

Revision Checklist – Renal Medicine   69

Revision Index – Gastroenterology   70

Revision Index – Endocrinology   71

Revision Index – Renal Medicine   72

PASTEST REVISION BOOKS FOR MRCP 1

PasTest are the leading independent specialists in postgraduate medical education. We publish a wide range of revision books including:

MCQs in Basic Medical Sciences for MRCP 1
> 300 exam-based MCQs with correct answers and detailed explanatory notes

MRCP 1 Practice Exams: 2nd edition
> Five complete MCQ Papers (300 MCQs) covering favourite Royal College topics

MRCP 1 MCQ Revision Book: 3rd edition
> 300 MCQs arranged by subject with correct answers and teaching notes, plus one complete mock exam

MRCP 1 Past Topics: A Revision Syllabus
> Contains authoritative lists of past topics which have occurred in the Royal College examination over the past 5 years

Explanations to the RCP Past Papers
> Correct answers and teaching notes related to the Royal College Green and Blue books of actual past exam questions

MRCP Part 1 MCQ Pocket Books
> Each pocket-sized book contains 100 MCQs on favourite Membership topics

Oxford Textbook of Medicine MCQs: 3rd edition
> 375 new MCQs related to the 1995 Oxford Textbook of Medicine and ideal for subject based revision

For full details of all our revision books contact PasTest today on **01565 755226** for a free copy of our current book catalogue and price list. Books sent by return of post worldwide.

For full details contact:
> **PasTest, Egerton Court, Parkgate Estate,**
> **Knutsford, Cheshire WA16 8DX**
> **Telephone 01565 755226 Fax 01565 650264**

INTRODUCTION

PasTest's MRCP Part 1 Pocket Books are designed to help the busy examination candidate to make the most of every opportunity to revise. With this little book in your pocket, it is the work of a moment to open it, choose a question, decide upon your answers and then check the answer on the back of the page. Revising "on the run" in this manner is both reassuring (if your answer is correct) and stimulating (if you find any gaps in your knowledge).

Each book contains 100 exam-based MCQs arranged by subject. Each author is a subject specialist who has based his selection of questions on past Royal College papers, and questions have also been designed specifically to address the basic sciences topics which have increasing prominence in the examination.

Each question consists of an initial statement followed by five possible completions, ABCDE. There is no restriction on the number of true or false items in a question. It is possible for all items in a question to be true or for all to be false. The four most important points of technique are:

1. Read the question carefully and be sure you understand it.
2. Mark your response clearly, correctly and accurately.
3. Use reasoning to work out your answer, but if you do not know the answer and cannot work it out, indicate "don't know".
4. The best possible way to obtain a good mark is to have as wide a knowledge as possible of the topics being tested in the examination.

It is possible to improve your mark by educated guessing, but this must be done with great care as incorrect answers are given a mark of −1 in the exam. You can use the books in this series to work out whether or not you are a good guesser by making a special mark against the responses that you have guessed before you check whether your responses are correct.

To get the best value from this book you should commit yourself to an answer for each item before you check the correct answer. With the answers on the back of each page, it can be tempting to find out which answers are correct before you have really decided on your own answer. But it is only by being sure of your own responses that you can ascertain which questions you would find difficult in the examination. Use the check boxes to mark your answers, or mark the parts of a question that you found difficult so that next time you look at the question you will be able to home in on your own personal areas of difficulty.

Books like the ones in this series, which consist of MCQs in subject categories, can help you to home in on specific topics and to isolate your weaknesses. You should plan a revision timetable to help you spread your time fairly over the range of subjects likely to appear in the examination. PasTest's *MRCP Part 1 Past Topics: A Revision Syllabus* will help you to work out which subjects deserve most of your revision time.

An effective revision plan should also include opportunities to practice your exam technique. Books of MCQ Practice Exams are indispensable and you should make time to sit at least two or three complete practice papers under timed conditions before the day of the actual examination arrives.

PasTest Revision Courses for MRCP 1
For 25 years PasTest, the leading independent specialists in post-graduate medical education, have been delivering top quality courses which have helped many thousands of doctors to pass the demanding MRCP Part 1 examination.

Our six-day MRCP Part 1 revision courses run three times each year at a convenient central London venue. Each delegate receives detailed course notes consisting of approximately 250 pages of exam-based MCQs with answers and comprehensive notes, plus many explanatory handouts.

> ✓ Learn from experienced and talented tutors with up-to-date knowledge of the requirements of the exam
>
> ✓ Teaching sessions focus on "favourite" exam topics and highlight possible areas of difficulty
>
> ✓ Four full practice exams enable you to constantly monitor your performance as the course progresses

For full details of the range of PasTest books and courses available for MRCP Part 1 candidates, contact PasTest today:

PasTest, Egerton Court, Parkgate Estate,
Knutsford, Cheshire WA16 8DX
Telephone: 01565 755226 Fax: 01565 650264

GASTROENTEROLOGY

Mark your answers with a tick (True) or a cross (False) in the box provided. Leave the box blank for 'Don't know'.

1. The hormone gastrin

- ☐ A is the main stimulus for acid secretion
- ☐ B has a plasma half-life of one hour
- ☐ C exerts its acid secretory effects by direct action on the parietal cell
- ☐ D has trophic effects on gastric mucosal endocrine cells
- ☐ E is found only in G cells of the gastric antrum

2. In primary biliary cirrhosis

- ☐ A positive antimitochondrial antibodies occur in over 95% of patients
- ☐ B pruritus may be the only clinical feature
- ☐ C centri-zonal necrosis is characteristic on liver biopsy
- ☐ D liver copper is increased
- ☐ E there is an association with Sjögren's syndrome

3. Following a large paracetamol overdose

- ☐ A the serum albumin is a reliable indicator of the severity of liver injury
- ☐ B alkalosis is a common feature
- ☐ C a prothrombin time of >100 seconds requires immediate treatment with vitamin K
- ☐ D liver transplantation should be considered when the serum bilirubin is >100 mmol/l
- ☐ E intravenous N-acetyl cysteine is the treatment of choice

Answers overleaf

1. D

Acid secretion in response to a meal has three phases, cephalic, gastric and duodenal. The main stimulus for acid secretion is neuronal, predominantly vagal cholinergic neurons. Gastrin is released from antral G cells and acts indirectly on the parietal cell via histamine released from ECL cells. In addition to stimulating release of histamine from ECL cells, gastrin also has a trophic action on these cells. Gastrin is also found in neurons of the central nervous system, although its function is unknown.

2. A B D E

Over 95% of patients with primary biliary cirrhosis have positive serum antimitochondrial antibodies, although they are not specific for primary biliary cirrhosis since positive results occur in some other liver diseases. Excess liver accumulation of copper accompanies the cholestasis, but is not usually sufficient to cause confusion with Wilson's disease. Centri-zonal necrosis is not a feature. Associated conditions include rheumatoid arthritis, scleroderma, Sjögren's syndrome, pancreatic atrophy and renal tubular acidosis.

3. E

Acute massive hepatocellular necrosis following paracetamol usually produces acidosis early on. Early referral for transplant assessment should be considered when pH falls below 7.31 and either the prothrombin time is >100 seconds or the plasma creatinine is >300 mmol/l. Serum albumin has a plasma half life of 14–16 days and is no indication of hepatocellular damage in the acute setting. Similarly bilirubin takes days to accumulate and jaundice is a late feature, often not appearing until fulminant hepatic failure is obvious. Intravenous N-acetyl cysteine is the treatment of choice and should be commenced as soon as possible after presentation.

4. Pernicious anaemia

- ☐ A is associated with gastric carcinoid tumours
- ☐ B is best diagnosed by positive intrinsic factor antibodies
- ☐ C is always associated with chronic atrophic gastritis
- ☐ D patients require regular endoscopic surveillance
- ☐ E is associated with an increased risk of carcinoma of the oesophagus

5. Bleeding oesophageal varices

- ☐ A may occur in the absence of cirrhosis
- ☐ B prognosis depends on the severity of the underlying liver disease
- ☐ C can be treated by transjugular intrahepatic portosystemic shunting
- ☐ D require immediate endoscopy and sclerotherapy
- ☐ E rarely respond to octreotide

6. The long acting somatostatin analogue octreotide

- ☐ A delays gastric emptying
- ☐ B reduces splanchnic arterial blood flow
- ☐ C constricts coronary arterioles
- ☐ D can only be given intravenously
- ☐ E may cause diarrhoea

Answers overleaf

4. A C

Chronic atrophic gastritis is an autoimmune inflammation centred on the parietal cell, often present for years before pernicious anaemia develops. The standard diagnostic test remains the Shilling test. The resulting achlorhydria leads to hypergastrinaemia, which in some patients induces mucosal endocrine cell hyperplasia, benign endocrine cell polyps and rarely, gastric carcinoid tumours. Endoscopic surveillance is of unproven benefit, but a single endoscopy at diagnosis may be of value in detection of early adenocarcinoma, present in approximately 5% of patients at diagnosis.

5. A B C

Whilst cirrhosis and portal hypertension are the commonest causes of variceal haemorrhage, any cause of portal hypertension will result in varices e.g. portal vein thrombosis or compression. Prognosis depends on the severity of the underlying liver disease. Endoscopy to confirm the diagnosis and attempt to prevent further blood loss by oesophageal banding or sclerotherapy should be performed after resuscitation. Intravenous octreotide is effective treatment in arresting haemorrhage and is as effective as sclerotherapy in continuous bleeding.

6. A B

Octreotide delays gastric emptying and decreases splanchnic arterial blood flow thereby reducing portal venous blood loss by limiting mesenteric blood flow. It also decreases small intestinal secretions and prolongs transit and may be given subcutaneously to control high stoma output in patients with an ileostomy. Unlike its predecessors, vasopressin and glypressin, it has no effect on coronary arterioles.

7. **In colorectal cancer**

   ☐ A there is a correlation between the consumption of meat and animal fat and the likelihood of developing colon cancer

   ☐ B faecal occult blood testing will detect 90% of cases

   ☐ C there is an increased incidence of rectal tumours in beer drinkers

   ☐ D the adenomatous polyposis coli (APC) gene maps to chromosome 2

   ☐ E hereditary non-polyposis colon cancer accounts for up to a third of all cases of colon cancer

8. **Chronic intestinal pseudo-obstruction may be a manifestation of**

   ☐ A small cell lung carcinoma

   ☐ B sarcoidosis

   ☐ C Parkinson's disease

   ☐ D lead poisoning

   ☐ E hyperthyroidism

9. **Recognised gastrointestinal infections in AIDS include**

   ☐ A cytomegalovirus

   ☐ B *Cryptococcus neoformans*

   ☐ C herpes simplex virus

   ☐ D *Pneumocystis carinii*

   ☐ E atypical mycobacteria

Answers overleaf

7. **A**

Epidemiological studies have shown that a diet high in animal fat and low in fruit and vegetable fibre predisposes to colon cancer. Familial adenomatous polyposis coli (FAPC) is an uncommon disorder, inherited in autosomal dominant manner and inevitably results in colon cancer. It accounts for approximately 1% of all cases. The FAPC gene is located on chromosome 5. In contrast, hereditary non-polyposiscolorrectal cancer (HNPCC) is relatively common accounting for up to 15% of cases of colon cancer. The familial colorectal cancer gene is linked to chromosome 2 and is also dominantly inherited. Faecal occult blood testing is a sensitive test for gastointestinal blood loss but its sensitivity and specifity is too low for it to be of value in the detection of colon cancer.

8. **A C D**

Other causes include diabetes, hypothyroidism, amyloidosis, chronic phenothiazine treatment, progressive systemic sclerosis and phaeo-chromocytoma.

9. **A C E**

Intestinal infection in the acquired immunodeficiency syndrome is common. In the oesophagus, herpes simplex, *Candida albicans* or cytomegalovirus may be the causative agent. Opportunistic small bowel disease occurs with cryptosporidium, *Isospora belli*, other sporing protozoa or atypical mycobacteria such as *Myobacterium avium* and *M. intracellulare* mimicking Whipple's disease. Colitis may be due to herpes simplex or cytomegalovirus. Gastrointestinal Kaposi's sarcoma may be the initial presentation of AIDS. *Cryptococcus neoformans* usually causes a meningitis and *Pneumocystis* a pneumonia.

10. *Helicobacter pylori*

- ☐ A is a Gram-positive spirochaete
- ☐ B has a prevalence that decreases with age
- ☐ C is associated with gastric carcinoma
- ☐ D can be diagnosed by a hydrogen breath test
- ☐ E produces the enzyme urease

11. Coeliac disease

- ☐ A is associated with HLA B12
- ☐ B is characterised by increased polymorphs in the lamina propria
- ☐ C is a cause of reversible male infertility
- ☐ D produces reduced small intestinal villus and crypt length
- ☐ E is associated with epilepsy

12. Hepatocellular carcinoma

- ☐ A is commoner in men
- ☐ B is uncommon following hepatitis C
- ☐ C may present as an acute abdomen
- ☐ D is associated with primary polycythaemia
- ☐ E rarely produces hepatomegaly

Answers overleaf

10. C E

H. pylori is a Gram-negative *Campylobacter*-like organism that survives in the mucous layer of the gastric mucosa close to the epithelium. Its prevalence increases with age and the presence of the organism can be diagnosed by the urease breath test, the bacteria producing urease which breaks down ingested C13-labelled urea to ammonia and carbon dioxide which can be detected in exhaled air. The presence of *H. pylori* carries a 6-fold increased risk for the development of gastric carcinoma.

11. C E

Coeliac disease is associated with HLA B8 and DR3. Dietary exposure to gluten results in intestinal inflammation most severe in the jejunum. Histologically there is a lymphocytic infiltrate in the lamina propria together with increased intraepithelial lymphocytes. Whilst villus height is lost, crypt length is increased reflecting increased cell turnover. Coeliac disease is associated with a number of neurological syndromes including epilepsy, and reversible infertility has been described in both men and women.

12. A C

Hepatocellular carcinoma is commoner in men and is associated with cirrhosis of any cause although it may occur in an otherwise histologically normal liver. Hepatomegaly is common and spontaneous rupture of the characteristically vascular tumour may lead to an acute presentation, and is a relative contraindication to liver biopsy. Hepatocellular carcinoma is one of a number of tumours that causes secondary polycythaemia.

13. Pseudomembranous colitis

- ☐ A typically spares the rectum
- ☐ B may occur after treatment with metronidazole
- ☐ C is caused by toxin-producing *Clostridium difficile*
- ☐ D is best treated with intravenous vancomycin
- ☐ E relapse is very uncommon after treatment

14. Chronic pancreatitis

- ☐ A may be caused by hypercalcaemia
- ☐ B rarely produces biliary strictures
- ☐ C is associated with peripheral vascular disease
- ☐ D may cause portal hypertension
- ☐ E is usually painless

15. Folic acid

- ☐ A is absorbed predominantly in the jejunum
- ☐ B blood levels are reduced in stagnant loop syndrome
- ☐ C bioavailability is impaired by cooking
- ☐ D body stores are adequate for 3 years
- ☐ E is effective treatment for alcohol-induced macrocytosis

Answers overleaf

13. B C

Pseudomembranous colitis describes the development of colonic inflammation in association with the use of antimicrobial drugs. Clindamycin was the antibiotic initially associated with this condition, but many broad spectrum antibiotics are now implicated. The cause is infection with a toxin-producing strain of *Clostridium difficile*. Multiple raised yellowish-white plaques are seen predominantly in the distal colon, although on rare occasions the rectum is spared. *C. difficile*, but not the toxin, may be found in the stools of 3% of normal adults and up to 50% of healthy neonates. Treatment is with oral vancomycin, oral or intravenous metronidazole or oral bacitracin. Relapse occurs in up to 33% of cases.

14. A C D

Pain is a prominent clinical feature in the majority of patients early on, but pain may lessen as the disease progresses and may disappear completely with end stage disease. Less commonly, patients may present with malabsorption without pain. Portal hypertension may be a result of peripancreatic fibrosis and compression of the portal vein. Although overt jaundice is relatively unknown, biliary strictures occur in >30% of patients with chronic pancreatitis.

15. A C

Folic acid is found in liver, nuts and green vegetables but is degraded by cooking. Absorption of the daily requirement of 100–200 µg occurs in the duodenum and jejunum. Body stores are sufficient for 4 months. Causes of folate malabsorption include coeliac disease, tropical sprue, jejunal and gastric resection, intestinal lymphoma, and drugs particularly methotrexate and sulphasalazine. In stagnant loop syndrome, folic acid is synthesised by bacteria and blood concentrations are increased. Alcoholic macrocytosis does not respond to folate supplementation.

16. Hepatic encephalopathy may be precipitated by

- ☐ A metabolic alkalosis
- ☐ B therapeutic paracentesis
- ☐ C treatment with omeprazole
- ☐ D intravenous normal saline
- ☐ E intravenous salt poor albumin

17. Hepatitis C

- ☐ A is an RNA virus
- ☐ B is more likely to produce jaundice than hepatitis B
- ☐ C is associated with hepatocellular carcinoma
- ☐ D infection may be complicated by hepatitis D
- ☐ E is more likely to result in cirrhosis than hepatitis B

18. The following are features of hepatic encephalopathy without coma:

- ☐ A inversion of normal sleep pattern
- ☐ B hyporeflexia
- ☐ C decreased muscle tone
- ☐ D constructional apraxia
- ☐ E absent pupillary response

19. The solitary rectal ulcer syndrome

- ☐ A is common in homosexual men
- ☐ B may cause iron deficiency anaemia
- ☐ C is associated with laxative abuse
- ☐ D usually involves an ulcer on the posterior rectal wall
- ☐ E commonly causes perineal pain

Answers overleaf

16. A B C D

Encephalopathy following therapeutic paracentesis is usually reversible and is uncommon. Its development is unrelated to the type of plasma expander used. Intravenous saline predisposes cirrhotic patients to fluid retention and ascites, and to encephalopathy from the resulting hyponatraemia and hypokalaemia.

17. A C E

Hepatitis C is an RNA flavivirus. It is less likely to produce jaundice than hepatitis B but a greater percentage of those infected will have chronic active hepatitis that will progress to cirrhosis, perhaps taking 20 years or more. Hepatocellular carcinoma is well recognised. Hepatitis D only complicates infection with hepatitis B.

18. A D

Constructional apraxia, inversion of normal sleep pattern, flapping tremor, hepatic foetor and personality disturbances are all well recognised clinical features of hepatic encephalopathy. In addition, brisk tendon reflexes, increased muscle tone and rigidity are common clinical findings. Pupillary responses are preserved.

19. B E

The solitary rectal ulcer syndrome is most common in women in their third decade. It is associated with constipation and disordered defaecation due to perineal descent and anterior rectal prolapse. Trauma and or ischaemia of the anterior rectal wall leads to ulceration, with approximately 80% of all ulcers being sited here. Perineal pain, soiling, mucous discharge and rectal bleeding are common symptoms, the latter leading to iron deficiency anaemia in some cases.

20. Cholecystokinin

- ☐ A relaxes smooth muscle
- ☐ B delays gastric emptying
- ☐ C stimulates gastric acid output
- ☐ D stimulates pancreatic exocrine secretion
- ☐ E increases appetite

21. Drug induced acute hepatitis may occur following treatment with

- ☐ A tetracycline
- ☐ B indomethacin
- ☐ C vitamin A
- ☐ D rifampicin
- ☐ E carbamazepine

22. The irritable bowel syndrome

- ☐ A is associated with disordered REM sleep
- ☐ B can be precipitated by travellers' diarrhoea
- ☐ C is characterised by visceral hypersensitivity
- ☐ D is associated with dysmenorrhoea
- ☐ E is characterised by rapid small intestinal transit

23. Wilson's disease is associated with

- ☐ A isolated psychiatric illness
- ☐ B increased biliary copper excretion
- ☐ C cerebellar ataxia
- ☐ D decreased serum caeruloplasmin
- ☐ E copper deposits in Descemet's membrane

Answers overleaf

20. B C D

The main physiological actions of cholecystokinin are to stimulate gall bladder contraction and pancreatic exocrine secretion. Its direct effect on smooth muscle is to cause contraction but it acts via a vagal reflex to produce fundal relaxation and hence delayed gastric emptying. Cholecystokinin has been extensively studied as a potential mediator of satiety.

21. B D E

Tetracycline produces steatosis. Vitamin A excess results in hepatic fibrosis. The commonest drugs causing an acute hepatitis are isoniazid, rifampicin, methyldopa, ketoconazole, verapamil, atenolol and tenplopril. Indomethacin and carbamazepine are quite rare causes.

22. B C D

Although the irritable bowel syndrome (IBS) is believed to represent disordered intestinal smooth muscle function, no characteristic abnormality of intestinal motility has been demonstrated. A lowered threshold to intraluminal distension is a common finding and reflects a heightened sensitivity. Other organs may also be involved, dysmenorrhoea, dysuria and urinary frequency being common associations. IBS can be precipitated by travellers' diarrhoea only in those subjects with a pre-existing affective disorder.

23. A E

Wilson's disease is a rare inherited disorder of copper metabolism characterised by failure of biliary excretion of copper. There is an accumulation of copper within the liver, decreased serum caeruloplasmin and accumulation of copper in the brain, predominantly the basal ganglia. Neurological manifestations include isolated psychiatric illness and more commonly a Parkinsonian movement disorder. Copper deposits also appear in Descemet's membrane close to the limbus of the cornea – Kayser-Fleischer rings.

24. Bilirubin

☐ A is entirely formed from haemoglobin breakdown

☐ B is transported in the blood bound to serum albumin before liver conjugation

☐ C is predominantly conjugated in the blood of normal subjects

☐ D is water soluble when conjugated

☐ E is metabolised to urobilinogen by gut bacterial action

25. Gastrointestinal manifestations of mutations of the *c-ret* oncogene include

☐ A sporadic gastric carcinoid tumours

☐ B Zollinger-Ellison syndrome

☐ C Hirschsprung's disease

☐ D cystic fibrosis

☐ E haemochromatosis

26. Gastro-oesophageal reflux

☐ A is characterised by increased oesophageal clearance

☐ B is best diagnosed by endoscopy

☐ C is most effectively treated by H_2-antagonists

☐ D occurs commonly in systemic sclerosis

☐ E rarely produces odynophagia

Answers overleaf

24. B D E

Bilirubin is formed from haem, but only 70% from haemoglobin, the remainder coming from non-erythroid haem and haemoproteins often in the liver. Unconjugated bilirubin, which makes up virtually all the serum bilirubin in normal subjects, is water insoluble, and therefore is transported to the liver bound to serum albumin. In the liver it is conjugated with glucuronic acid to increase water solubility and facilitate excretion. In the gut it is metabolised by gut bacteria to urobilinogen which undergoes an enterohepatic circulation.

25. C

The *c-ret* oncogene codes for a tyrosine kinase which is normally expressed in the embryo in developing neuroendocrine cells of the gastrointestinal tract and elsewhere. Mutation may therefore lead to failure of normal developmental migration of intestinal neurons leading to Hirschsprung's disease, or predisposition to neuroendocrine tumours. Hence mutations of the *c-ret* oncogene also account for the MEN syndromes 2 A and B. The gene for MEN 1, which includes Zollinger-Ellison syndrome and the gene for haemochromatosis have not yet been cloned and that for cystic fibrosis codes for the cystic fibrosis transmembrane conductance regulator.

26. D

Patients with gastro-oesophageal reflux disease (GORD) usually reflux acid into their distal oesophagus. The resulting acid-induced damage produces mucosal inflammation and also may reduce oesophageal clearance which improves with successful treatment. Oesophageal clearance may however be of primary aetiological significance as in systemic sclerosis, where poor clearance prolongs exposure to acid. Odynophagia is a characteristic symptom of GORD, which is most accurately diagnosed by 24 hour pH monitoring. For acid reflux, proton pump inhibitors with or without a prokinetic provide the best symptomatic relief.

27. Recognised side effects of treatment with omeprazole include

- ☐ A gynaecomastia
- ☐ B erythema multiforme
- ☐ C headache
- ☐ D bradycardia
- ☐ E pancreatitis

28. Systemic sclerosis of the gastrointestinal tract

- ☐ A most commonly affects the oesophagus
- ☐ B is associated with primary biliary cirrhosis
- ☐ C causes narrowing of the small intestinal lumen
- ☐ D may produce diarrhoea responding to antibiotic therapy
- ☐ E is a recognised cause of steatorrhoea

29. Complications of total parenteral nutrition (TPN) include

- ☐ A cholestasis
- ☐ B hyperlipidaemia
- ☐ C pancreatitis
- ☐ D aspiration pneumonia
- ☐ E acute renal failure

30. Dietary fat

- ☐ A is ingested primarily as cholesterol
- ☐ B can only be absorbed as free fatty acid
- ☐ C stimulates cholecystokinin release from the small intestine
- ☐ D absorption is enhanced by bile salts
- ☐ E decreases small intestinal transit time

Answers overleaf

27. A B C

Gynaecomastia occurs rarely with omeprazole and is more commonly seen with H_2-antagonist treatment. Severe headache is probably the commonest reason for discontinuing omeprazole therapy. Bradycardia, occasionally due to atrioventricular block, and pancreatitis have not yet been reported with omeprazole but both are recognised side effects of H_2-antagonist treatment.

28. A B D E

The gastrointestinal tract is frequently affected in systemic sclerosis with the oesophagus being involved in up to 80% of patients. Abnormalities are best seen by manometry and include low resting oesophageal pressure and non-progressive contractions. Symptoms include heartburn, dysphagia for liquids and solids and pulmonary aspiration on lying down. Stomach involvement is rare, but systemic sclerosis causes dilatation and stasis of the small intestine and delayed transit. Abdominal pain, distension, diarrhoea and steatorrhoea, which is probably due to bacterial overgrowth, may occur. Colonic symptoms are uncommon. Systemic sclerosis is associated with autoimmune disease such as primary biliary cirrhosis and the CREST syndrome.

29. A B

Chronic cholestasis rarely progressing to liver failure is a recognised complication of TPN but the underlying pathophysiology is poorly understood. Hyperlipidaemia is also recognised and is easily correctable. Aspiration pneumonia is a complication of enteral nutritional support, and severe pancreatitis is an indication for TPN.

30. C D

Ingested fat is predominantly triglyceride and is broken down by pancreatic lipase to free fatty acids or monoglyceride. Fatty acid stimulates cholecystokinin release from mucosal endocrine cells of the small intestine resulting in gallbladder contraction and delivery of bile salts to the intestine. Bile salts aid micelle formation by emulsification with fatty acids and monoglyceride which are then absorbed. Any unabsorbed fat reaching the distal small intestine slows intestinal transit, a reflex termed the ileal brake.

31. Mesalazine compounds

- ☐ A are useful in the maintenance of remission of ulcerative colitis
- ☐ B have no value in the treatment of active small bowel Crohn's disease
- ☐ C are contraindicated in pregnancy
- ☐ D may cause impotence
- ☐ E can be given by enema

32. Delayed gastric emptying

- ☐ A occurs in hyperglycaemia
- ☐ B is characteristic of functional dyspepsia
- ☐ C may be treated with erythromycin
- ☐ D may be caused by anti-Parkinsonian drugs
- ☐ E is a feature of the dumping syndrome

33. *Clostridium difficile*

- ☐ A produces a cytopathic toxin detectable in >90% of patients with pseudomembranous colitis
- ☐ B is part of the normal colonic flora in 15% of healthy adults
- ☐ C is the cause of up to a third of all cases of antibiotic related diarrhoea
- ☐ D is best treated with intravenous vancomycin
- ☐ E may cause toxic dilatation of the colon

Answers overleaf

31. A E

The use of mesalazine to maintain remission in ulcerative colitis is well established. More recently high doses of slow-release mesalazine have been shown to be effective in the treatment of active small bowel Crohn's disease. Generally 5-acetylsalicylic acid compounds are safe in pregnancy and do not produce impotence, although sulphasalazine causes oligospermia, a side effect attributable to its sulphapyridine moiety. Acetylsalicylic acid foam enemas are now available as effective treatment for colitis of the rectosigmoid colon.

32. A C D

The delayed gastric emptying seen in diabetic patients with gastroparesis can be effectively treated by the motilin receptor agonist erythromycin. Gastroparesis may affect diabetic control and hyperglycaemia contributes to the delayed gastric emptying by reducing vagal tone to the stomach. Anti-Parkinsonian drugs by merit of their anti-cholinergic and or dopaminergic effects also slow gastric emptying. No consistent gastric motility disorder has been identified in functional dyspepsia although 50% of patients may show delayed gastric emptying.

33. A C E

C. difficile can be found as part of the normal colonic flora in about 3% of healthy adults. Its toxin is detectable in nearly all patients with pseudomembranous colitis and in up to 33% of those with less severe antibiotic related diarrhoea. Presentation varies from self-limiting diarrhoea to fulminating colitis with toxic dilatation. First line therapy should be oral metronidazole and if this fails oral vancomycin, but both may be given intravenously if necessary.

ENDOCRINOLOGY

Mark your answers with a tick (True) or a cross (False) in the box provided. Leave the box blank for 'Don't know'.

34. The close anatomical relations of the pituitary fossa include
- ☐ A the cavernous sinus
- ☐ B the internal carotid artery
- ☐ C the third cranial nerve
- ☐ D the sphenoidal sinus
- ☐ E the eighth cranial nerve

35. Craniopharyngioma
- ☐ A rarely presents in adulthood
- ☐ B may cause diabetes insipidus without anterior pituitary failure
- ☐ C may cause optic atrophy
- ☐ D rarely recurs after surgery in adults
- ☐ E is associated with suprasellar calcification

36. The following are true of insulin-like growth factor-1 (IGF-1):
- ☐ A the site of IGF-1 synthesis is unknown
- ☐ B serum levels are low in acromegaly
- ☐ C serum levels are low in starvation
- ☐ D its serum concentration is ten-fold lower than insulin
- ☐ E there is a single specific IGF binding protein in serum

Answers overleaf

34. A B C D

A number of important structures lie close to the pituitary fossa and can be encroached upon by an expanding pituitary tumour. Immediately lateral to the fossa (which does not have bony lateral walls) lies the cavernous sinus, through which runs the sixth cranial nerve. The third, fourth and upper two divisions of the fifth cranial nerves lie in the lateral wall of the sinus. The internal carotid artery lies in the sinus lateral to the dorsum sella, its siphon fitting under the 'shoulder' of the dorsum. The fossa is an indentation in the roof of the sphenoidal sinus, which may be invaded by downward growth of a pituitary tumour.

35. B C E

Although craniopharyngiomas arise from embryonic remnants (Rathke's pouch), they not infrequently present for the first time in adulthood. Unlike true pituitary tumours, they arise above the pituitary fossa and therefore can damage the hypothalamus (and ADH secreting neurones) without compressing the pituitary causing diabetes insipidus, and disturbances of sleep, appetite and temperature regulation. Downward expansion may cause chiasmatic or optic nerve compression. The tumour is typically cystic, calcified in 35% of adult cases and although never malignant, is almost impossible to excise completely, responds poorly to radiotherapy and may require repeated cyst drainage.

36. C

IGF-1 (previously known as somatomedin C) is produced predominantly in the liver in response to circulating growth hormone (GH) and mediates the majority of the growth promoting actions of GH. Unlike GH, it has a long plasma half-life and hence a random raised serum level is a useful diagnostic indicator of acromegaly. Levels fall rapidly during illness and starvation. IGF circulates at concentrations 1000 times higher than that of insulin and can cross react with the insulin receptor but binding to six different IGF binding proteins (to which insulin does not bind) prevents this *in vivo*. Within tissues, enzymes are secreted which cleave the binding proteins releasing the IGF-1 to act as a growth factor locally.

37. Growth hormone (GH) secretion is stimulated by

- ☐ A somatostatin
- ☐ B glucose
- ☐ C amino acids
- ☐ D hexapeptides related to metenkephalins
- ☐ E sleep

38. In hypopituitarism

- ☐ A selective gonadotrophin deficiency may be present
- ☐ B concomitant diabetes insipidus (DI) may be masked by anterior pituitary failure
- ☐ C adrenal steroid replacement must be started before thyroid replacement
- ☐ D mineralocorticoid replacement is usually necessary
- ☐ E in men, androgen replacement will cause masculinisation and restore fertility

39. In active acromegaly

- ☐ A treatment is not necessary for a small intrasellar tumour which is not expanding
- ☐ B external beam radiotherapy will normalise growth hormone (GH) levels in most cases within 6 months
- ☐ C transphenoidal surgical removal is the treatment of choice for large tumours causing visual field constriction
- ☐ D bromocriptine will normalise GH levels in over 90% of cases
- ☐ E somatostatin analogues can achieve clinical and biochemical remission

Answers overleaf

37. C D E

Glucose, as in the glucose tolerance test, suppresses GH levels. Failure to suppress in this test is used to diagnose acromegaly. Somatostatin and dopamine agonists also suppress GH secretion and are used therapeutically in acromegaly. GH secretion is pulsatile with increased frequency and amplitude of 'spikes' during sleep, exercise and stress. Additional stimulators of GH release include hypoglycaemia (as in insulin tolerance test), glucagon, amino acids such as arginine and lysine (as in Bovril), hypothalamic GH-releasing hormone (GHRH) and a newly identified range of synthetic hexapeptides (hexarelin, GH releasing peptides or GHRPs) derived from the structure of meten-kephalin, all of which have been used in tests for GH deficiency.

38. A B C

Isolated deficiencies of gonadotrophins or growth hormone are well described and may be due to failure of secretion of their respective hypothalamic releasing hormones. Concomitant cortisol deficiency reduces the severity of and may even conceal diabetes insipidus, possibly because it lowers glomerular filtration rate. DI may therefore be revealed by adrenal replacement therapy. In combined adrenal and thyroid failure, an adrenal crisis may be precipitated by starting thyroxine replacement therapy before corticosteroids. Aldosterone synthesis and secretion occur in the zona glomerulosa of the adrenal cortex and are largely ACTH-independent. Mineralocorticoid deficiency sufficient to require replacement therapy is therefore rare in hypopituitarism. Fertility depends on the gonadotrophins, which must be replaced for fertility to be achieved.

39. E

Active acromegaly doubles mortality at all ages (due to associated hypertension, diabetes and atheroma) and should therefore be treated in all but the elderly or very frail. GH levels fall relatively slowly after external beam radiotherapy and are normalised in only 40% of cases at 2 years after treatment; interim medical treatment may be necessary. Large extrasellar tumours, especially those compressing the optic chiasma, should be treated surgically; the transfrontal route must be used to allow adequate access. Bromocriptine normalises GH in only about 30% of cases. Long-acting somatostatin analogues can suppress GH levels and cause resolution of acromegaly, and may be effective in some cases which are unresponsive to bromocriptine.

40. Acromegaly

☐ A is rarely caused by a pituitary tumour larger than 1 cm

☐ B is best diagnosed by a fasting GH level

☐ C is not associated with elevations in other pituitary hormones

☐ D may be associated with kidney stones

☐ E is associated with colonic polyps

41. Antidiuretic hormone (ADH)

☐ A is synthesised in the posterior pituitary

☐ B is a cyclic octapeptide

☐ C circulates in the blood stream bound to neurophysin

☐ D is released by carbamazepine

☐ E is released by ethanol

42. The following are true of diabetes insipidus (DI):

☐ A serum sodium is typically above 140 mmol/l

☐ B it may be caused by lithium

☐ C the congenital nephrogenic form shows autosomal dominant inheritance

☐ D the nephrogenic form may be aggravated by thiazide diuretics

☐ E in the central form (cranial DI), vasopressin replacement is essential for survival

Answers overleaf

40. D E

Growth hormone secreting (somatotroph) pituitary tumours are almost always macroadenomas (>1cm) and frequently expand beyond the sella. Random GH levels are of no use in diagnosing acromegaly as levels taken during a 'spike' will be raised in normal people (see Q37). Somatotroph tumours often co-secrete or immuno-stain for prolactin as well as GH and over 80% co-secrete the alpha subunit of the glycoprotein hormones. Associated features of acromegaly include sleep apnoea, multiple skin tags, adenomatous polyps and hypercalcuria causing renal stones due to a direct renal tubular action of GH. The presence of hypercalcaemia suggests hyperparathyroidism associated with multiple endocrine neoplasia (MEN) 1 syndrome.

41. B D

ADH is a nonapeptide synthesised in neurones in the hypothalamus (mostly the supraoptic and paraventricular nuclei). It is transported (bound to neurophysin carrier proteins) along axons descending the pituitary stalk to the posterior pituitary, where it is released into the circulation. Its release is stimulated by high plasma osmolality, hypovolaemia, smoking and by many drugs including morphine, chlorpropamide and carbamazepine (the last two are used to treat partial cranial diabetes insipidus). ADH secretion is suppressed by naloxone, phenytoin and ethanol.

42. A B E

Deficiency of antidiuretic hormone (central DI) or impaired action on the kidney collecting ducts (nephrogenic DI) causes polydypsia and polyuria resulting in dehydration. With a normal thirst mechanism, treatment is not essential. Urinary fluid losses can be compensated for by drinking more although the serum remains slightly concentrated (raised sodium concentration, typically >140 mmol/l). The nephro-genic form may be caused by drugs such as lithium, hypercalcaemia, hypokalaemia, intrinsic renal disease (e.g. polycystic kidneys) or be inherited as an X-linked trait.

43. Galactorrhoea

- [ ] A is often caused by antidepressants
- [ ] B may be caused by anti-emetics
- [ ] C should prompt a search for occult malignancy
- [ ] D is associated with chronic liver disease
- [ ] E is most commonly due to a pituitary microadenoma in women

44. In anorexia nervosa

- [ ] A loss of pubic hair occurs
- [ ] B patients may present with primary amenorrhoea
- [ ] C luteinizing hormone (LH) levels are elevated
- [ ] D the erythrocyte sedimentation rate (ESR) is high
- [ ] E cortisol levels are low

45. In females with hirsutism

- [ ] A circulating free testosterone levels are usually increased
- [ ] B endometriosis is a common cause
- [ ] C cliteromegaly is common
- [ ] D late-onset congenital adrenal hyperplasia may be a cause
- [ ] E there may be associated insulin resistance

Answers overleaf

43. B E

Galactorrhoea is invariably due to hyperprolactinaemia or an increased sensitivity of the breast to prolactin. Prolactin secretion is under dominant negative control by dopamine from the hypothalamus and hence hypothalamic damage or dopamine antagonists such as the major tranquillisers and anti-emetics (e.g. metoclopramide) cause hyperprolactinaemia. Anti-depressants have little anti-dopaminergic action and rarely cause significant increases in prolactin. Hyperprolactinaemia and galactorrhoea occur independently of gynaecomastia which is due to raised oestrogen levels (e.g. from drugs, tumours or liver disease). Prolactin microadenomas (<1 cm) are the commonest cause of galactorrhoea in women. Prolactin levels are also raised in pregnancy, by stress and by raised TRH levels in primary hypothyroidism.

44. B

Anorexia nervosa is associated with a number of endocrine abnormalities, most apparently due to malnutrition or weight loss. These include low gonadotrophin levels with loss of the normal pulsatile pattern of secretion (a profile typical of prepubertal girls), high-normal or supranormal cortisol levels (possibly related to depression), and high growth hormone levels (possibly due to reduced negative feedback on the pituitary by low circulating levels of insulin-like growth factors). The eating disorder and weight loss may begin before menarche and so prevent pubertal gonadotrophin release and the appearance of puberty itself. An elevated ESR suggests organic disease (the ESR is normal or low in anorexia), whereas loss of pubic hair suggests hypopituitarism (in anorexia, pubic hair is conserved and fine, dark lanugo hair may appear on the body and face).

45. A D E

Hirsutism (increased androgen dependent hair growth) affects up to 20% of women. In over 95% of cases it is due to increased ovarian androgen production with mildly raised free testosterone levels, often associated with oligomenorrhoea, polycystic ovaries, obesity and a degree of insulin-resistance (polycystic ovary syndrome, PCOS). Cliteromegaly is rare, indicates true virilisation (along with breast atrophy and voice change) and should prompt a search for other causes such as an ovarian or adrenal tumour, or congenital adrenal hyperplasia (CAH). So-called 'late-onset CAH' usually results from relatively conservative mutations in the 21-hydroxylase gene and produces a phenotype indistinguishable from PCOS.

46. The following statements are true:

☐ A levels of sex-hormone binding globulin are increased in Klinefelter's syndrome

☐ B hypogonadotrophic hypogonadism may be associated with anosmia

☐ C there is a high risk of seminoma in the testicular feminisation syndrome

☐ D azoospermia is invariable in Klinefelter's syndrome

☐ E Klinefelter's syndrome causes hypogonadotrophic hypogonadism

47. In Graves' disease

☐ A the eye signs usually improve when hyperthyroidism is controlled by antithyroid drugs

☐ B levels of thyroid-stimulating hormone (TSH) are normal

☐ C neonatal hyperthyroidism may result from transplacental passage of maternal thyroxine

☐ D the thyroid is stimulated by antimicrosomal antibodies

☐ E amenorrhoea may occur

48. Features of primary autoimmune hypothyroidism include

☐ A increased incidence of type 1 diabetes and Addison's disease

☐ B pretibial myxoedema

☐ C multiple serous effusions

☐ D ataxia

☐ E paranoia and delusions

46. A B C E

Circulating testosterone is mainly bound to sex-hormone binding globulin, the levels of which are generally inversely related to prevailing testosterone concentrations. Hypogonadotrophic hypogonadism may be associated with impaired or absent sense of smell (Kallman's syndrome). In the testicular feminisation syndrome the gonads are undescended testes (intra-abdominal or in the inguinal canal) and are therefore at increased risk of malignancy. Typical 47,XXY individuals with Klinefelter's syndrome often show complete seminiferous tubule dysgenesis and therefore azoospermia, but others (especially mosaics) may be relatively well masculinised and rare cases have produced spermatozoa. Klinefelter's syndrome is the commonest cause of bilateral testicular failure resulting in hypogonadism with raised FSH/LH (hypergonadotrophic). It is not inherited but caused by chromosomal non-dysjunction in the sperm/ova or, rarely, post-fertilisation (3% of cases).

47. E

In Graves' disease, thyroid stimulation is due to activation of the TSH receptors by autoantibodies which develop against the receptor. By contrast, autoantibodies directed against other thyroid components (e.g. microsomes of the follicular cells or thyroglobulin) cause damage rather than stimulation of the gland. Elevated thyroxine and tri-iodothyronine levels act through negative feedback on the hypothalamus and pituitary to reduce secretion of TSH, the circulating levels of which are suppressed to below the normal range. Thyroid eye disease is often temporally separated from the hyperthyroidism. Amenorrhoea is a recognised feature of thyrotoxicosis of any cause. Neonatal hyperthyroidism results from IgG TSH-receptor-stimulating antibodies which cross the placenta and stimulate the fetal thyroid; it resolves spontaneously after some weeks when the antibodies are cleared from the circulation. Only a small amount of maternal thyroxine crosses the placenta.

48. A C D E

Autoimmune thyroid failure is associated with other organ-specific autoimmune disease; the combination with Addison's disease is referred to as 'Schmidt's syndrome'. Pericardial and pleural effusions and ascites, reversible with thyroid replacement, may occur. Rare neurological complications include bilateral cerebellar damage and 'myxoedema madness' (first described by Richard Asher), which includes hallucinations, agitation, delusions and paranoia. Localised 'myxoedema' consisting of cutaneous hyaluronic acid deposits and most often appearing on the shins, is a feature of Graves' disease.

49. Thyrotoxicosis

- ☐ A with a markedly raised ESR suggests subacute (de Quervain's) thyroiditis
- ☐ B without a raised thyroidal radioiodine uptake may occur after pregnancy
- ☐ C is best treated with surgery
- ☐ D may cause diarrhoea
- ☐ E may cause intermittent muscle paralysis

50. The following statements are true:

- ☐ A total thyroxine levels rise in normal pregnancy
- ☐ B TSH levels are low in hyperemesis gravidarum
- ☐ C amiodarone may cause hyper- or hypothyroidism
- ☐ D hypothyroidism may develop during treatment with interferon alpha
- ☐ E free T3 and T4 levels fall in acute illness but TSH rises

51. The following are true of G-proteins:

- ☐ A they are involved in intracellular signalling via cyclic AMP
- ☐ B they hydrolyse ATP when activated
- ☐ C activating mutations may cause growth hormone secreting pituitary tumours
- ☐ D activating mutations are seen in multiple endocrine neoplasia syndrome Type II
- ☐ E inactivating mutations may cause pseudohypoparathyroidism

Answers overleaf

49. A B D E

Self-limiting thyrotoxicosis due to discharge of stored hormone (often followed by transient hypothyroidism) is seen in de Quervain's post-viral thyroiditis associated with a raised ESR. Iodine uptake into the thyroid is low and new thyroid hormone synthesis is suppressed. A similar pattern of self-limiting thyroid disturbance may be seen in the postpartum period, so-called postpartum thyroiditis, believed to be of autoimmune origin. Treatment in either case is symptomatic with beta blockers. Carbimazole is ineffective. In thyrotoxicosis of any cause, surgery is reserved for refractory or non-compliant cases. Diarrhoea, proximal muscle weakness, leucopenia and rarely periodic muscle paralysis (especially in Chinese) are manifestations of thyrotoxicosis.

50. A B C D

Over 99% of circulating T4 is bound to plasma proteins, mainly thyroid-binding globulin (TBG) but also pre-albumin and albumin. Oestrogen raises TBG levels (e.g. pregnancy, oral contraceptive) and hence total thyroxine concentrations. Congenitally low or high TBG levels may occur and nephrotic syndrome may lower TBG along with other serum proteins. High hCG levels in early pregnancy and especially hyperemesis gravidarum cross-react with the TSH receptor causing mild hyperthyroidism with low TSH. The high iodine content of amiodarone may cause hyper- or hypothyroidism. Treatment with cytokines such as interferons or interleukin-2 may precipitate or exacerbate autoimmune hypothyroidism. In acute illness, the syndrome of 'sick euthyroidism' is seen with rapid falls in free T3 followed by reduced levels of TSH and free T4.

51. A C E

Membrane G proteins mediate signalling via cyclic AMP by linking surface membrane receptors for certain glycoprotein hormones (e.g. GHRH, TSH, ACTH, glucagon, catecholamines) to the adenylate cyclase enzyme that generates cyclic AMP. They are so-called because they hydrolyse GTP on activation. Inhibitory G proteins (Gi) mediate suppression of adenylate cyclase by somatostatin. G protein mutations that cause constitutive adenylate cyclase activation have been found in growth hormone pituitary tumours, thyroid tumours and precocious puberty associated with McCune Albright syndrome. Mutations that prevent cyclic AMP generation impair parathyroid hormone action in pseudohypoparathyroidism.

52. In the investigation of Cushing's syndrome

☐ A 24 hour urine free cortisol collection is a first line investigation

☐ B ACTH levels in the normal range suggest an adrenal tumour

☐ C a rise in ACTH levels following an injection of corticotrophin releasing hormone (CRH) suggests a pituitary tumour

☐ D MRI scanning of the pituitary is the best investigation to differentiate ectopic ACTH production from pituitary dependent disease (Cushing's disease)

☐ E plasma cortisol is characteristically suppressed following high doses of dexamethasone (8 mg/day) in Cushing's syndrome due to ectopic ACTH production

53. Common features of Cushing's syndrome due to adrenal carcinoma include

☐ A retarded growth in children

☐ B clitoromegaly

☐ C subconjunctival oedema

☐ D marked hyperpigmentation

☐ E supraclavicular fat pads

54. Atrial natriuretic peptide (ANP)

☐ A is synthesised in the juxtaglomerular apparatus of the kidney

☐ B is released in response to hypervolaemia

☐ C promotes sodium retention in the renal tubule

☐ D is itself a vasoconstrictor

☐ E induces salt craving

Answers overleaf

52. A C

If hypercortisolism (Cushing's syndrome) is suspected, first line investigations include 24 hour urine free cortisol collection and morning and midnight serum cortisols to confirm loss of diurnal variation. Additionally overnight or low dose dexamethasone suppression tests may be performed. Patients with depression or alcoholism may demonstrate abnormal results with all these tests and are best evaluated after abstinence from alcohol and off all neuroleptic drugs. Once hypercortisolism is confirmed, the site of overactivity – adrenal, pituitary or ectopic production of CRF or ACTH – must be determined. A suppressed ACTH level is characteristic of an adrenal source. If ACTH is detectable in the serum, suppression of steroid levels with high dose dexamethasone, an increase in ACTH after CRH stimulation and higher ACTH levels on inferior petrosal sinus sampling than in the peripheral blood suggest a pituitary tumour rather than ectopic ACTH production. MRI scanning of the pituitary is an unreliable test alone as ACTH secreting pituitary tumours are often too small to detect (< 3 mm) and up to 25% of normal people have small inactive pituitary microadenomas of no relevance.

53. A B C E

Features of cortisol excess in Cushing's syndrome due to all causes include central fat deposition (including the round 'moon', face, 'buffalo' hump and supraclavicular fat pads), subconjunctival oedema (a useful physical sign) and growth retardation or arrest in children. Functional adrenal tumours (both benign adenoma and carcinoma) often produce excess androgen and/or oestrogen in addition to cortisol; marked masculinisation (including clitoromegaly) or feminisation therefore suggests an adrenal tumour rather than pituitary-driven Cushing's disease, in which excess sex steroid production is rare. Primary adrenal over-production of cortisol suppresses ACTH secretion; very high ACTH levels and pronounced hyperpigmentation suggest that Cushing's syndrome is driven by an 'ectopic' source of ACTH such as a lung or pancreatic carcinoid.

54. B

ANP is a 28 amino-acid peptide synthesised by the myocytes of the right atrium and ventricle and released in response to volume overload as detected by increased right atrial stretch. It corrects the hypervolaemia by effects which oppose those of angiotensin and aldosterone: increasing renal sodium excretion, vasodilatation, reducing thirst and salt craving as well as inhibiting the actions of renin, aldosterone and ADH. Its true physiological importance remains unclear.

55. The following features suggest inadequate glucocorticoid replacement in Addison's disease:

- ☐ A insomnia
- ☐ B tiredness
- ☐ C loss of appetite
- ☐ D hypokalaemia
- ☐ E total daily hydrocortisone dosage of 10 mg

56. Causes of hypokalaemia with increased plasma renin activity include

- ☐ A psychogenic vomiting
- ☐ B laxative abuse
- ☐ C Conn's syndrome
- ☐ D diuretic abuse
- ☐ E syndrome of apparent mineralocorticoid excess (11-betahydroxysteroid dehydrogenase deficiency)

57. In congenital adrenal hyperplasia (CAH)

- ☐ A 21-hydroxylase deficiency is the commonest variety
- ☐ B virilisation may be prevented by glucocorticoid treatment
- ☐ C adrenal crisis may occur within a few days of birth
- ☐ D blood 17-hydroxyprogesterone concentrations are greatly increased
- ☐ E severe hypoglycaemia may occur

Answers overleaf

55. B C

Individual requirements for glucocorticoid replacement vary widely: some patients require as little as 5 mg/day whereas others may need 30 mg/day. Symptoms suggestive of inadequate replacement include tiredness, loss of energy, anorexia, vomiting, headache and 'flu-like' malaise; postural hypotension, hyperkalaemia and an elevated blood urea concentration may also be present. Insomnia may be due to over-replacement or to taking the evening dose too late. Other features of overdosage include excessive weight gain (especially if with oedema or Cushingoid features), hypertension and hypokalaemia.

56. A B D

All the factors listed cause hypokalaemia and total body potassium depletion which may be profound and symptomatic. The important differential diagnosis is from Conn's syndrome, in which primary adrenal overproduction of aldosterone increases sodium–potassium exchange in the distal tubule, causing sodium retention (leading to hypertension) and excessive urinary potassium losses. In primary hyperaldosteronism, plasma renin activity is suppressed by sodium and water overload, as is also the case with carbenoxolone, a steroidal compound with similar sodium-retaining and potassium-losing effects. The membrane bound enzyme 11-betahydroxysteroid dehydrogenase metabolises cortisol but not aldosterone and hence normally protects the mineralocorticoid receptor from stimulation by cortisol. Deficiency of this enzyme activity causes the syndrome of apparent mineralo-corticoid excess. Although hypokalaemia occurs in this syndrome the renin-angiotensin-aldosterone system is suppressed. In conditions A, B and D, sodium and water losses and the resulting intravascular volume depletion stimulate plasma renin activity.

57. A B C D E

CAH is a group of diseases due to inherited deficiencies of various steroid biosynthetic enzymes, of which 21-hydroxylase is the most commonly affected. The manifestations of CAH depend on the site of the enzyme defect and on the relative effects of 'upstream' precursor excesses and of end-product deficiency. Cortisol deficiency may be severe and fatal in the neonatal period. With 21-hydroxylase defects, 17-hydroxyprogesterone and androgenic steroids accumulate, caus-ing virilisation. Glucocorticoid treatment not only replaces cortisol but also suppresses androgenic precursors, and can prevent virilism; 17-hydroxyprogesterone and testosterone levels are useful guides to adjusting dosage. Life-threatening hypoglycaemia may accompany cortisol deficiency due to intercurrent illness or omission of steroids.

58. In hypercalcaemia

- ☐ A serum alkaline phosphatase is always elevated in primary hyperparathyroidism
- ☐ B malignancy can be a cause in the absence of bone metastases
- ☐ C severe hypocalcaemia may follow removal of a single parathyroid adenoma
- ☐ D detectable parathyroid hormone (PTH) levels indicate hyperparathyroidism and the need for surgical treatment
- ☐ E peritoneal dialysis is effective in severe cases

59. Idiopathic hypoparathyroidism is associated with

- ☐ A increased incidence of Addison's disease
- ☐ B chronic mucocutaneous candidiasis
- ☐ C basal ganglia calcification, commonly causing Parkinsonism
- ☐ D short fourth and fifth metacarpals
- ☐ E good response of hypocalcaemia to calcium and vitamin D treatment

Answers overleaf

58. B C E

95% of hypercalcaemia is due to hyperparathyroidism or malignancy. Serum alkaline phosphatase levels are only raised in hyperparathyroidism in severe disease. Squamous cell, renal and breast tumours may produce parathyroid hormone related peptide (a different gene from parathyroid hormone itself) and hence 'humoral' hypercalcaemia in the absence of metastases. Suppressed parathyroid hormone (PTH) production by the remaining three parathyroid glands in parathyroid adenoma may result in temporary (days to weeks) but severe hypocalcaemia following adenoma removal. Detectable PTH levels with modern assays in the presence of hypercalcaemia do indicate hyperparathyroidism; however, surgery is only indicated if symptoms are present, there is renal impairment or serum calcium exceeds 3.0 mmol/l. Treatment of hypercalcaemia includes aggressive rehydration, calcitonin (acutely), bisphosphonates (in malignancy), surgery (in hyperparathyroidism) and dialysis in refractory cases.

59. A B E

Hypoparathyroidism may be due to autoimmune disease, when autoantibodies are often directed against several tissues and may produce clinical disease including hypothyroidism, Addison's disease, type 1 diabetes, primary ovarian failure and pernicious anaemia. Chronic mucocutaneous candidiasis is common in hypoparathyroidism associated with autoimmune disease and in Di George syndrome. Calcification of the basal ganglia occurs in both hypoparathyroidism and pseudohypoparathyroidism (which is due to target organ resistance to parathyroid hormone, not to parathyroid failure), but is rarely associated with Parkinsonism. Several somatic features (including short stature, 'moon-face' and short metacarpals and metatarsals) occur in pseudohypoparathyroidism, but not in true hypoparathyroidism. Both hypoparathyroidism and pseudohypoparathyroidism are treated with calcium supplements and vitamin D derivatives such as alfacalcidol; parathyroid hormone is not currently available for practical therapeutic use.

60. In osteoporosis

- ☐ A thyrotoxicosis may be a cause
- ☐ B serum alkaline phosphatase may be raised above normal levels
- ☐ C serum osteocalcin is a marker of bone formation
- ☐ D treatment with bisphosphonates may prevent vertebral fractures
- ☐ E bone density should be monitored at 6 monthly intervals in severe disease

61. The following statements are true of Paget's disease:

- ☐ A hydroxycholecalciferol is a useful treatment
- ☐ B it is believed to be primarily a disease of osteoblasts
- ☐ C deafness may occur
- ☐ D serum alkaline phosphatase levels reflect disease activity
- ☐ E extensive disease on bone scan is an indication for treatment

62. Features of the multiple endocrine neoplasia (MEN) syndrome type 1 include

- ☐ A parathyroid hyperplasia
- ☐ B multiple neuromata around the eyes and mouth
- ☐ C acromegaly
- ☐ D medullary carcinoma of the thyroid
- ☐ E profuse watery diarrhoea

Answers overleaf

60. A C D

Osteoporosis is most commonly age-related and/or post-menopausal. Other causes include hypogonadism, thyrotoxicosis, steroid excess, immobility, myeloma, rheumatoid arthritis, phenytoin and heparin. Bone density is reduced to less than 2.5 standard deviation units below that of healthy young subjects. There are no biochemical markers which fall outside the normal range, although bone formation (indicated by serum osteocalcin, alkaline phosphatase and urinary procollagen peptides) must be lower than the rate of bone resorption (indicated by urinary hydroxyproline or pyridinium–collagen crosslinks). Treatment with bisphosphonates, either cyclical etidronate or alendronate (continuously), have been shown to increase bone density and reduce vertebral fractures. Bone density is best measured by dual energy X-ray absorptiometry (DEXA) but the inaccuracy is such that significant changes can usually only be detected over 1–2 years.

61. C D

Paget's disease is believed to be primarily an osteoclast disorder, although coupled increases in osteoblast activity are required for new bone formation. Disease activity is indicated by urinary hydroxyproline or pyridinium–collagen crosslinks but serum alkaline phosphatase is often the simplest indicator. Complications include pain, bone/skull deformity, deafness, paraplegia, high-output cardiac failure, pathological fracture and osteosarcoma. Radiological evidence of extensive disease alone is insufficient indication for treatment. Effective treatments are calcitonin, mithramycin and bisphosphonates, the last being currently the most common choice.

62. A C E

The MEN 1 syndrome comprises two or more of the following: para-thyroid tumours (hyperplasia is commoner than adenoma, and carcinoma is very rare), pituitary tumours, and pancreatic endocrine tumours. The latter include insulinoma, glucagonoma, gastrinoma, carcinoid, VIPoma (causing the Verner–Morrison syndrome of watery diarrhoea, hypo-kalaemia and achlorhydria) and rare tumours producing growth hormone releasing hormone, which can cause acromegaly. Medullary carcinoma of the thyroid, phaeochromocytoma and parathyroid tumours define the MEN-2 syndrome; multiple facial neuromata (especially of the eyelids, tongue and lips) occur in a variant of MEN-2 syndrome, previously classified as 2B and now described separately as MEN-3. MEN-2A has been linked to the *ret* proto-oncogene in chromosome 10.

63. In the differential diagnosis of hypoglycaemia

- ☐ A high C-peptide concentrations in the presence of hypoglycaemia suggest factitious insulin administration
- ☐ B a high ratio of proinsulin to insulin in a fasting blood sample is a feature of insulinoma
- ☐ C nesidioblastosis should be considered in the neonate or infant
- ☐ D the tolbutamide test is useful in the diagnosis of insulinoma
- ☐ E a 72-hour fast fails to produce hypoglycaemia in up to 20% of insulinomas

64. The following statements are true:

- ☐ A growth hormone deficiency in adults produces no effects
- ☐ B magnesium is excreted in both urine and faeces
- ☐ C steroid receptors are present at the cell surface
- ☐ D steroid receptors can bind to DNA
- ☐ E thyroid hormone receptors can bind to DNA

Answers overleaf

63. B C

In both normal and neoplastic β-cells, proinsulin is cleaved enzymatically to produce equimolar amounts of insulin and C-peptide. Hypoglycaemia caused by exogenous insulin (which contains virtually no C-peptide) inhibits pancreatic insulin release and circulating C-peptide levels are therefore low. In insulinomas, defective post-translational processing of proinsulin may allow proinsulin to be secreted in addition to insulin and C-peptide. Virtually all patients with an insulinoma will become hypoglycaemic (venous plasma glucose concentration 3.5 mmol/l) and neuroglycopenic during a 72-hour fast. The tolbutamide test is dangerous and now obsolete. Nesidioblastosis is diffuse β-cell hyperplasia occurring throughout the pancreas, in contrast to the focal β-cell proliferation of insulinomas. Although rare, it is a common cause of hyperinsulinaemia and hypoglycaemia in early childhood, when discrete insulinomas are rare.

64. B D E

Recently a syndrome of growth hormone deficiency in adults has been described comprising lack of energy, low mood, decreased muscle and increased fat mass and possibly reduced myocardial function, osteoporosis and hypercholesterolaemia. Who should receive expensive growth hormone replacement therapy remains controversial. Magnesium is lost in both urine (increased in diabetes, alcohol excess, hypercalcaemia, renal failure diuretic, amphotericin aminoglycoside, cisplatin and cyclosporin treatment) and faeces (increased with diarrhoea). Steroids, vitamin D and thyroxine all act via intracellular (cytoplasmic) receptors which after hormone binding migrate to the nucleus and bind directly to DNA. All other hormones act via cell surface receptors.

65. Phaeochromocytoma

- ☐ A is excluded by a normal CT scan of the adrenals
- ☐ B may secrete dopamine
- ☐ C is associated with islet-cell tumours
- ☐ D pending surgery, should be treated by β-blockade
- ☐ E may be localised on an IVP

66. The following statements are true:

- ☐ A calcitonin-gene related peptide has a potent calcium-lowering effect
- ☐ B diarrhoea is common in the gastrinoma syndrome
- ☐ C DDAVP is a powerful vasoconstrictor
- ☐ D thromboembolic disease is common in the glucagonoma syndrome
- ☐ E high gastrin levels are associated with pernicious anaemia

Answers overleaf

65. B E

Ten per cent of phaeochromocytomas lie outside the adrenal medulla, and even those in the classical site may not be detected by CT scan. The presence of large tumours may be deduced from displacement of the renal outline on an IVP. In addition to adrenaline (which predominates in adrenal phaeochromocytomas) and noradrenaline (extra-adrenal tumours), dopamine may be secreted, especially by malignant tumours. Phaeochromocytomas occur in association with medullary carcinoma of the thyroid and parathyroid tumours (MEN-2), but not with pancreatic endocrine or pituitary tumours (MEN-1). Treatment with β-blockers alone is hazardous: removal of β-adrenergic vasodilation in skeletal muscle may cause a hypertensive crisis. Treatment should therefore start with an α-blocker (e.g. phenoxybenzamine), to which a β-blocker may be added to control tachycardia.

66. B D E

Calcitonin-gene related peptide is a peptide encoded within the calcitonin gene complex, but with entirely different actions. It has no effect on calcium metabolism but is a powerful vasodilator. Secretory diarrhoea occurs in most patients with gastrinoma and is mainly due to acid hypersecretion. DDAVP is an analogue of arginine vasopressin which, unlike the native peptide has virtually no vasoconstrictor activity and can therefore be used in patients with ischaemic heart disease. Gastrin release is inhibited by the presence of acid in the stomach; reduced acid secretion (as in the atrophic gastritis of pernicious anaemia) therefore stimulates gastrin secretion.

RENAL MEDICINE

Mark your answers with a tick (True) or a cross (False) in the box provided. Leave the box blank for 'Don't know'.

67. The following can cause acute renal failure in overdose:
- ☐ A paracetamol
- ☐ B paraquat
- ☑ C indomethacin
- ☑ D ethylene glycol
- ☐ E iron

68. Useful measurements to distinguish between acute renal failure and chronic renal failure include
- ☐ A sodium level in urine
- ☑ B ultrasound scan of kidneys to assess size
- ☑ C serum phosphate
- ☑ D presence of left ventricular hypertrophy on ECG
- ☐ E hypokalaemia

69. Characteristics of the hepatorenal syndrome include
- ☑ A intratubular deposition of bilirubin
- ☐ B oliguria
- ☐ C daily urinary sodium losses exceeding 50 mmol
- ☑ D good prognosis following renal transplantation
- ☐ E diuresis following albumin infusion

67. A B C D E

Paracetamol and iron overdose can both cause ATN as will indomethacin. ATN is also seen in ethylene glycol poisoning with the associated histological hallmark of intratubular calcium oxylate crystals. Paraquat causes death in 50% of patients who swallow it and acute renal failure and pulmonary fibrosis are major features of poisoning.

68. B D

Urinary sodium excretion may be a useful parameter to distinguish pre-renal uraemia from established ATN. However the main abnormalities that indicate chronic renal disease are small renal size, evidence of long-standing hypertension, established bone disease and normocytic anaemia.

69. B

The hepatorenal syndrome results from reduced cortical perfusion secondary to the accumulation of vasoactive substances thought to be either endotoxin or an interleukin, which are normally cleared in the liver. Oliguria and a daily urine sodium excretion of under 10 mmol are the rule. The syndrome only resolves if there is a dramatic improvement in hepatic function and so liver transplantation is the treatment of choice. Interestingly, the kidneys of a patient with hepatorenal syndrome will function if transplanted into a recipient with a normal liver. Although the blood volume is frequently low, plasma expanders rarely improve renal function.

70. In patients with acute renal failure

☐ A eosinophilia and hypocomplementaemia are typical of allergic interstitial nephritis

☐ B non-oliguria indicates a better prognosis

☐ C dopamine typically causes diuresis

☑ D renal obstruction is excluded by polyuria

☐ E aminoglycosides are always contraindicated and should be avoided if at all possible

71. In the normal kidney

☐ A maximal tubular re-absorption of phosphate can be increased physiologically

☐ B tubular re-absorption of phosphate can be increased by PTH

☐ C in chronic acidosis the excretion of ammonium in the urine is greater than in acute acidosis

☐ D alkalosis leads to decreased secretion of potassium

☐ E acetazolamide leads to decreased distal secretion of potassium

72. Renal excretion of water is increased in association with

☐ A hyperkalaemia

☐ B hypokalaemia

☐ C recovery phase of ATN

☐ D hyperaldosteronism

☐ E chronic renal failure

Answers overleaf

70. B

Acute allergic interstitial nephritis is not characteristically associated with hypocomplementaemia; a low serum complement and eosinophilia would suggest atheroembolic disease. Non-oliguric patients usually have less severe renal failure and have a better prognosis. Although dopamine at a dose of 2–5 µg/kg/min may increase renal blood flow this is not necessarily accompanied by a diuresis. Intermittent or partial obstruction both cause nephrogenic diabetes insipidus and may also cause salt wasting.

71. A C

Phosphate homoeostasis is influenced by dietary phosphate intake and its re-absorption can be increased when phosphate intake is diminished; the action of PTH leads to phosphaturia. Alkalosis results in kaliuresis, and acetazolamide inhibits both hydrogen ion excretion and bicarbonate re-absorption, leading to acidosis and increased potassium secretion by the distal tubule.

72. B C E

Acquired nephrogenic diabetes insipidus is commonly associated with diseases that primarily affect the renal medulla. These include hypokalaemic interstitial nephritis and the recovery phase of ATN. One of the first symptoms of chronic renal failure may be nocturia, which is again due to collecting tubule insensitivity to ADH and the osmotic diuretic effect of raised blood urea.

73. Filtration at the glomerulus

- ☐ A results from a net filtration pressure of 10 mm Hg in normal subjects
- ☐ B is favoured if a molecule is positively charged
- ☐ C results in a filtration fraction of 40% in normal subjects
- ☐ D results in the formation of approximately 360 litres of filtrate per day in normal man
- ☐ E is reduced by efferent arteriolar constriction

74. Concerning the renal function at 36 weeks of pregnancy

- ☐ A a serum creatinine of 150 μmol/l requires investigation
- ☐ B a urea of 1 mmol/l is due to malnutrition
- ☐ C there is a reduced glomerular filtration rate
- ☐ D the serum magnesium concentration is typically low
- ☐ E uric acid levels are characteristically high

75. The clearance

- ☐ A of a substance by the kidney is defined as the volume of blood cleared of that substance in one minute
- ☐ B of a compound which is freely filtered by the kidney and neither secreted nor reabsorbed is a measure of the renal plasma flow
- ☐ C of inulin is normal when plasma inulin = 0.02 mg/ml, urinary inulin = 2.5 mg/ml, and the urinary flow rate = 60 ml/hr
- ☐ D of urea is an accurate estimate of the glomerular filtration rate (GMR) in the hydrated state
- ☐ E of penicillin is reduced by probenecid

Answers overleaf

73. A B

The pressure favouring filtration at the glomerulus = hydrostatic pressure − (oncotic pressure + Bowman's capsule pressure) = 45 − (25 + 10) = 10 mm Hg. The basement membrane consists of negatively charged glycoproteins (including sialic acid) and collagen. The filtration fraction = glomerular filtration rate (GFR) divided by renal plasma flow = 125/600 or 20% in normal man. Daily filtration is approximately 180 litres. Efferent arteriolar constriction increases the GFR and may be involved in the phenomenon of 'autoregulation' if renal perfusion pressure falls.

74. A D

Glomerular filtration rate increases considerably towards the end of the second trimester and during the third trimester of pregnancy and creatinine usually falls to the lower end of the normal range; this is also manifest by a very low blood urea. The serum concentrations of many nutrients are diminished including the minerals such as magnesium. Rising levels of uric acid in serum are significant and may indicate the onset of pre-eclampsia.

75. A C E

The definition of clearance is correct. The clearance of a substance freely filtered but not secreted or reabsorbed by the kidney (e.g. *inulin*) is an accurate estimate of GFR. Renal plasma flow is measured from the clearance of a compound which is filtered and secreted by the kidney (e.g. PAH).

The formula for inulin clearance = $\dfrac{U_{in} \times V}{P_{in}}$

where U_{in} and P_{in} are the concentrations of inulin in urine and plasma and V is the rate of urine flow/min. Clearance thus calculated is 125 ml/min and is a measurement of the normal GFR. Urea is reabsorbed by the kidney even in the hydrated state (approx. 40%) and the clearance is much lower than the GFR. Probenecid decreases tubular penicillin secretion and hence its renal clearance.

76. The following will result in an increase in urinary sodium excretion :

☐ A a decrease in renal sympathetic nervous activity

☐ B a rise of 15 mm Hg in renal arterial pressure

☐ C a 10% increase in glomerular filtration rate (GFR)

☐ D a decrease in the plasma protein concentration

☐ E an increase in venous volume

77. Ascent to 10,000 ft can lead to a reduction in arterial pCO_2 in normal people. The response in the kidney

☐ A leads to a fall in plasma $[HCO_3]^-$

☐ B is corrective rather than compensatory

☐ C results in arterial pCO_2 returning to normal

☐ D leads to a fall in plasma pH

☐ E occurs predominantly in the proximal tubules

78. Renin

☐ A is released from the cells of the macula densa in response to sodium depletion

☐ B release is stimulated by renal sympathetic nervous stimulation

☐ C increases in response to cortical ischaemia

☐ D leads to the production of a plasma borne vasoconstrictor

☐ E leads to an increase in thirst

Answers overleaf

76. A B D E

Despite the mechanism of 'autoregulation' which maintains renal blood flow and the GFR within narrow limits, small increases in the renal arterial pressure are paralleled by decreases in proximal sodium re-absorption and sodium excretion is increased. An increase in venous volume stimulates baroreceptors in the atria and in renal capillaries leading to increased sodium excretion by decreased proximal re-absorption and decreased sympathetic tone. Decreased plasma oncotic pressure reduces proximal sodium re-absorption.

77. A D E

The reduction in arterial pCO_2 will lower the plasma HCO_3 and increase pH (respiratory alkalosis). The increased pH will reduce the rate of H^+ secretion, less bicarbonate will be reabsorbed and a further fall in plasma HCO_3 will occur. This will correct the pH. The overall response is compensatory as arterial pCO_2 remains low and plasma HCO_3 is much reduced. The main site of bicarbonate re-absorption is proximal.

78. B C D E

Renin is a proteolytic enzyme found in the granular cells of the juxta-glomerular apparatus and produced in response to sodium depletion (detected by the cells of the macula densa) or to volume depletion (detected by the atrial and renal capillary baroreceptors). Reduced atrial stretch results in increased renal sympathetic tone and renin release. Renin acts on angiotensinogen (renin substrate) to produce angiotensin I which is converted to angiotensin II, a potent vasocon-strictor which also stimulates thirst. Redistribution of renal blood flow away from the outer cortex stimulates renin release, which may be of relevance to sodium retention in some disease states.

79. Relative contraindications to continuous ambulatory peritoneal dialysis (CAPD) include

☐ A obesity

☐ B rheumatoid arthritis

☐ C previous appendicectomy

☐ D chronic obstructive airways disease

☐ E cardiac failure

80. Indications for urgent dialysis in uraemic patients include

☐ A asterixis

☐ B itching

☐ C pericarditis

☐ D peripheral neuropathy

☐ E hiccoughing

81. A man of 40 is found to be uraemic. The following facts might give a useful lead to the aetiology:

☐ A he had haematuria in childhood

☐ B he works in an iron foundry

☐ C three of his children had haemolytic disease of the newborn

☐ D he has tablets regularly for fibrositis

☐ E he suffers from migraine

79. A B D

The CAPD dialysate contains glucose, the concentration of which varies according to the tonicity of the solution, and its absorption exacerbates obesity – catheter placement may be impossible in the obese patient. Previous abdominal surgery only contraindicates CAPD if adhesions or a potential infection risk such as a stoma or fistula are present. Diaphragmatic splinting with PD fluid can impair ventilation in the patient with chronic pulmonary disease, whereas patients with severe deformity may not possess the dexterity necessary to perform CAPD.

80. A C E

Asterixis and hiccoughing are signs of uraemic encephalopathy and so are indications for dialysis. Pericarditis is also life-threatening as cardiac tamponade may occur owing to bleeding from the inflamed pericardium. This may be exacerbated by anticoagulants used during haemodialysis and so reduced heparinization, regional heparinization of the extracorporeal circulation or peritoneal dialysis should be used. Itching is usually a manifestation of secondary hyperparathyroidism and may be worsened acutely during haemodialysis. Peripheral neuropathy seldom resolves even with intensive dialysis, but fortunately is rare nowadays.

81. A B D E

Chronic analgesic usage is associated with renal failure, as is retroperitoneal fibrosis due to methysergide treatment of migraine. Childhood haematuria may be indicative of a progressive glomerulonephritis or of familial renal disease e.g. Alport's syndrome. Chronic exposure to silica (foundry workers) can lead to heavy-metal type interstitial nephritis or glomerulosclerosis.

82. Renal failure is unusual in

- ☐ A carcinoma of the kidney
- ☐ B systemic lupus erythematosus
- ☐ C multiple myeloma
- ☐ D Wegener's granulomatosis
- ☐ E Paget's disease

83. In moderate (not end stage) chronic renal failure

- ☐ A the level of blood insulin is inappropriately high compared with the level of blood glucose
- ☐ B the main cause of growth failure is growth hormone deficiency
- ☐ C polyuria is more common than oliguria
- ☐ D typically there is hypercalciuria
- ☐ E treatment and control of hypertension will improve the glomerular filtration rate

84. A 35-year-old male with chronic renal failure due to focal glomerulosclerosis has a blood pressure of 170/100, a creatinine clearance of 40 ml/min and no oedema. Treatment should include

- ☐ A an ACE inhibitor
- ☐ B a low potassium diet
- ☐ C a low sodium diet
- ☐ D a low protein diet
- ☐ E fluid restriction and diuretics

Answers overleaf

82. A E

Although renal failure is fairly common in SLE and Wegener's granulomatosis, optimal immunosuppressant therapy and renal replacement greatly improve prognosis such that other co-morbidity may become dominant in determining the outcome. The prognosis of patients with myelomatous renal failure is poor, with a median survival of 20 months.

83. A C E

In chronic renal failure there is insulin resistance but urinary calcium excretion is very low. The loss of urinary concentrating ability is an early feature and polyuria may ensue. Metabolic acidosis is a major contributor to the growth retardation of childhood renal failure.

84. A C

Progression of moderate chronic renal failure can be attenuated by optimising hypertensive control especially with ACE inhibitors; protein restriction has little effect. Reducing sodium intake may also improve blood pressure control but diuretics have no effect upon outcome.

85. When imaging the renal tract of uraemic subjects

☐ A renal obstruction is best diagnosed by static radionuclide scanning

☐ B dehydration is indicated to improve the quality of intravenous urograms

☐ C lateral displacement of the ureters is characteristic of retroperitoneal fibrosis

☐ D large kidneys exclude a diagnosis of chronic renal failure

☐ E coarse kidney scarring is diagnostic of reflux nephropathy

86. In the haemolytic-uraemic syndrome

☐ A the prognosis is worse in those with diarrhoea

☐ B case to case transmission is frequent

☐ C *E. coli* 0157 is the commonest cause in the UK

☐ D fragmentation of red cells may occur

☐ E haemodialysis and peritoneal dialysis are equally effective

87. Rapidly progressive glomerulonephritis

☐ A may be precipitated by exposure to hydrocarbons

☐ B is always associated with antibodies to the glomerular basement membrane

☐ C is associated with haemoptysis most commonly in smokers

☐ D has a worse prognosis if the patient is anuric

☐ E may present with the nephrotic syndrome

Answers overleaf

85. None correct

The screening test for renal obstruction is ultrasound; if the collecting system is dilated, pressure studies may be needed to confirm the diagnosis. Dehydration may precipitate acute or chronic renal failure owing to contrast nephropathy especially in the elderly, arteriopaths, diabetics and patients with myeloma. The ureters are deviated medially in retroperitoneal fibrosis. Chronically diseased kidneys usually shrink but they characteristically remain large in diabetes, amyloidosis and polycystic kidney disease. Causes of coarse kidney scarring include reflux nephropathy, obstructive uropathy, papillary necrosis and renovascular disease.

86. B C D

Haemolytic-uraemic syndrome occurs either sporadically or in minor epidemics, the latter often associated with infective diarrhoea (including that due to verocytotoxin-producing coliforms) and having a better prognosis. The resulting oliguric acute renal failure is best treated by either haemodialysis or haemofiltration as hypercatabolism is often a feature.

87. A C D E

There is an increased incidence of prior exposure to volatile hydrocarbons in patients developing rapidly progressive glomerulonephritis. More than half of the patients have systemic vasculitis with or without anti-neutrophil cytoplasmic antibody (ANCA), and the remainder have anti-glomerular basement membrane disease, or other systemic disease such as cryoglobulinaemia, SLE or malignancy. Goodpasture's syndrome is more common in smokers. An acute nephritic onset is usual. Response to treatment is variable but less likely in anuric patients and those with anti-glomerular basement membrane disease.

88. Membranous glomerulonephritis

- ☐ A is characterised by highly selective proteinuria
- ☐ B usually leads to end-stage renal failure within 2 years
- ☐ C is characterised by IgG deposits within the basement membrane
- ☐ D commonly presents with the nephritic syndrome
- ☐ E is associated with malignancy

89. IgA nephropathy

- ☐ A is the most common form of glomerulonephritis
- ☐ B is complicated by end-stage renal failure in over 50% of those affected
- ☐ C may show glomerular crescents during episodes of macroscopic haematuria
- ☐ D causes loin pain owing to bleeding from peripheral renal arteries
- ☐ E has a worse prognosis when proteinuria exceeds 1 g/day

90. Nephrotic syndrome is associated with

- ☐ A cholesterol emboli
- ☐ B acute renal failure
- ☐ C venous thrombosis
- ☐ D hypokalaemia
- ☐ E pneumococcal infection

Answers overleaf

88. C E

Membranous glomerulonephritis usually presents with moderate to nephrotic range non-selective proteinuria, and granular IgG deposits are seen within the basement membrane of glomeruli. Approximately one third of patients develop end-stage renal failure but the course is usually over several years after diagnosis; adverse prognostic signs at presentation are hypertension and early renal impairment. There is an association with bronchial and gastrointestinal tract malignancy.

89. A C E

IgA nephropathy appears more common than other forms of glomerulonephritis, at least in Europe, North America and Australia. Only about 15–25% progress to end-stage renal failure; poor prognostic factors include uraemia at presentation, heavy proteinuria and frequent episodes of macroscopic haematuria. Acute exacerbations usually coincide with infections and are characterised histologically by glomerular crescents, and clinically by loin pain (owing to swelling of the kidney), macroscopic haematuria and heavy proteinuria. The loin pain–haematuria syndrome is a different disease, the aetiology of which is uncertain.

90. B C D E

Cholesterol emboli complicate atheromatous aorto-renovascular disease and are not associated with the hypercholesterolaemia of the nephrotic syndrome. Hypocomplementaemia and hypoglobulinaemia predispose to most bacterial infections, especially pneumococcal disease. Acute renal failure, due to ATN, may complicate the nephrotic syndrome if intravascular volume is severely depleted; hypokalaemia often accompanies loop diuretic therapy.

91. Renal vein thrombosis is a complication of

☐ A renal carcinoma

☐ B gastroenteritis in childhood

☐ C renal amyloidosis

☐ D IgA glomerulonephritis

☐ E pyelonephritis

92. In adult polycystic kidney disease

☐ A patients are always hypertensive

☐ B there may be cysts in the pancreas and the liver

☐ C haematuria is a recognised feature

☐ D transplantation is contraindicated

☐ E there is an association with medullary sponge kidney

93. Uraemic osteodystrophy is associated with

☐ A hyperparathyroidism

☐ B hyperphosphataemia

☐ C decreased 1,25 dihydroxycholecalciferol

☐ D increased osteoclastic activity within bone

☐ E increased calcium absorption from the gut

94. The following are genetically-transmitted diseases that may involve the kidney:

☐ A von Hippel-Lindau syndrome

☐ B cystinosis

☐ C vesico-ureteric reflux

☐ D Noonan's syndrome

☐ E systematic lupus erythematosus

Answers overleaf

91. A B C

Renal vein thrombosis is recognised in the nephrotic syndrome especially when this is due to membranous glomerulonephritis; it may complicate volume depletion in infants. Renal carcinoma can invade the renal veins, predisposing to thrombosis that can propagate into the inferior vena cava.

92. B C

Polycystic kidney disease is associated with hepatic cysts (in about 70% of cases) and also pancreatic cysts, although failure of the respective organs is rare. Berry aneurysms in the cerebral circulation occur in 25% of patients. Large or infected kidneys may need to be removed prior to transplantation.

93. A B C D

The major metabolic abnormalities in uraemic osteodystrophy include hyperparathyroidism (resulting in increased bony resorption), hyper-phosphataemia and decreased 1-alpha hydroxylation of vitamin D (such that calcium absorption from the gut is attenuated).

94. A B C

Von Hippel-Lindau syndrome is autosomal dominant and manifests as spinal and cerebellar haemangiomata, renal carcinomas and retinal angiomas. Vesico-ureteric reflux has a familial predisposition but cystinosis is a recessively inherited condition in which chronic renal failure, short stature, eye and cardiac disease are cardinal features. Noonan's syndrome involves a hereditary form of hyper-trophic cardiomyopathy with other, non-renal, syndromal associations.

95. Concerning vesico-ureteric reflux

☐ A it may remain clinically silent until adulthood

☐ B it may present with nausea and vomiting

☐ C it is usually associated with coliform urinary tract infection

☐ D ureteric reimplantation is of no value

☐ E the prophylactic antibiotic of choice is ampicillin

96. Active tuberculosis of the urinary tract

☐ A is a recognised cause of renal calculi

☐ B may cause ureteric obstruction when treated

☐ C is a contraindication to renal transplantation

☐ D is a recognised cause of urge incontinence

☐ E is associated with a normal chest X-ray in over 50% of cases

97. Diabetic microalbuminuria

☐ A occurs within 10 years of diabetes

☐ B is a predictor of early cardiovascular mortality in type II
diabetes

☐ C is best assessed by a timed collection during the day

☐ D is not affected by improved glycaemic control

☐ E when accompanied by hypertension is best treated with ACE
inhibitors

Answers overleaf

95. A B

Vesico-ureteric reflux often only presents as chronic renal failure in adult life; even at this stage ureteric reimplantation may be of benefit for symptomatic reflux. Evidence of urinary tract infection is only present in about 40% of cases.

96. A B C D E

Renal tuberculosis may present clinically or radiologically with calculous disease. Since healing is by fibrosis, lesions within the ureter may form strictures especially during the first six weeks of treatment. Active tuberculosis anywhere contraindicates renal transplantation. Transplant recipients with quiescent disease require continuous prophylaxis; isoniazid is preferred to rifampicin since the latter increases metabolism of cyclosporin A. Tuberculous cystitis may cause disabling frequency or dysuria necessitating urinary diversion or a bladder augmentation operation. There is no radiological sign of pulmonary tuberculosis in about 60% of cases.

97. B E

Microalbuminuria is the first manifestation of diabetic nephropathy, but it may not occur until the second to third decades after the diagnosis of diabetes. It is best assessed by examination of early morning urine specimens, as albumin excretion can vary diurnally. Albuminuria can be reduced by optimising glycaemic control and blood pressure; ACE inhibitor agents have been shown to be of particular benefit in the treatment of hypertension.

98. In distal (type 1) renal tubular acidosis

☐ A there is reduced ammonia formation despite good glomerular filtration rate

☐ B the urine pH cannot be below 7.0

☐ C there is an association with renal calcification

☐ D there is hypokalaemia

☐ E the condition only occurs in children

99. The following drugs may be harmful in patients with chronic renal failure:

☐ A oxytetracycline

☐ B mesalazine

☐ C omeprazole

☐ D felodipine

☐ E ibuprofen

100. Concerning the use of erythropoeitin in patients with end-stage renal failure

☐ A adequate haemoglobin response is anticipated within the first month

☐ B oral iron supplementation is sufficient to maintain the response

☐ C the response to intravenous administration is better than to the subcutaneous route

☐ D secondary hyperparathyroidism may reduce the haemoglobin response

☐ E haemodialysis and continuous ambulatory positoneal dialysis (CAPD) patients respond equally well

Answers overleaf

98. A C D

Classical distal renal tubular acidosis (type I) is due to a failure of hydrogen ion excretion into the urine and renal function is well preserved. Nephrocalcinosis or renal tract calculi occur in approximately 70% of cases and the patients have marked hypokalaemia. Typically the urinary pH is > 5.5 and often > 6.0 during acute acidosis. Acquired type I renal tubular acidosis is common with many renal medullary pathologies.

99. A B E

Tetracyclines (except doycycline) can exacerbate uraemia by increasing urea generation, whereas non-steroidal anti-inflammatory agents will reduce the glomerular filtration rate in patients with compromised renal perfusion (e.g. cardiac failure, elderly patients during intercurrent illness). The sulphonamide component of mesalazine can provoke interstitial nephritis.

100. D

Subcutaneous administration of erythropoeitin (EPO) is more efficacious than intravenous administration as the latter reduces bioavailability of the product. Initiation phase treatment may last 3–4 months before target haemoglobin is achieved, and response is enhanced by parenteral iron supplementation. The mean haemoglobin concentration of a haemodialysis population is usually less than that of a corresponding CAPD programme, perhaps due to increased blood losses, red cell fragmentation or comorbidity in the former group. Hyperparathyroidism and chronic infection also diminish response to EPO.

GASTROENTEROLOGY: REVISION CHECKLIST

Liver disease

- ☐ Jaundice
- ☐ Primary biliary cirrhosis
- ☐ Chronic liver disease
- ☐ Gilbert's syndrome
- ☐ Hepatic mass/sub-phrenic abscess

Small bowel disease/Malabsorption

- ☐ Coeliac disease
- ☐ Cholera toxin/ gastroenteritis
- ☐ Malabsorption
- ☐ Carcinoid syndrome
- ☐ Whipple's disease

  (See also Crohn's disease' below)

Large bowel disorders

- ☐ Ulcerative colitis/Crohn's disease
- ☐ Diarrhoea
- ☐ Irritable bowel syndrome
- ☐ Pseudomembranous colitis

Oesophageal disease

- ☐ Achalasia
- ☐ Dysphagia/oesophageal tumour
- ☐ Gastro-oesophageal reflux/tests
- ☐ Oesophageal chest pain

Stomach and pancreas

- ☐ Acute pancreatitis
- ☐ Gastric acid secretion
- ☐ Persistent vomiting
- ☐ Stomach cancer

Miscellaneous

- ☐ GI tract bleeding
- ☐ Abdominal X-ray
- ☐ GI hormones

ENDOCRINOLOGY: REVISION CHECKLIST

Diabetes and glycaemic control

- [ ] Diabetes
- [ ] Hypoglycaemia
- [ ] Hepatic gluconeogenesis
- [ ] Insulinoma

Adrenal disease

- [ ] Cushing's syndrome
- [ ] Congenital adrenal hyperplasia
- [ ] Addison's disease
- [ ] ACTH action

Thyroid/Parathyroid disease

- [ ] Action/metabolism of thyroxine
- [ ] PTH
- [ ] Calcitonin
- [ ] Graves' disease/ exophthalmos
- [ ] Hypothyroidism
- [ ] Thyroid cancer

Pituitary disease

- [ ] Acromegaly
- [ ] Chromophobe adenoma
- [ ] Hyperprolactinaemia
- [ ] Hypopituitarism
- [ ] Pituitary hormones

Miscellaneous

- [ ] SIADH
- [ ] Polycystic ovary syndrome/ infertility
- [ ] Hirsutism
- [ ] Short stature
- [ ] Sweating
- [ ] Weight gain

NEPHROLOGY: REVISION CHECKLIST

Nephrotic syndrome/related glomerulonephritis
- ☐ Nephrotic syndrome
- ☐ Membranous glomerulonephritis
- ☐ Minimal Change disease
- ☐ Renal vein thrombosis
- ☐ Hypocomplementaemia & glomerulonephritis
- ☐ SLE nephritis

Renal failure
- ☐ Acute versus chronic
- ☐ Chronic renal failure
- ☐ Acute renal failure
- ☐ Haemolytic-uraemic syndrome
- ☐ Rhabdomyolysis

Urinary abnormalities
- ☐ Macroscopic haematuria
- ☐ Discolouration of the urine
- ☐ Nocturia
- ☐ Polyuria

Basic renal physiology
- ☐ Normal renal physiology/function
- ☐ Water excretion/urinary concentration

Miscellaneous
- ☐ Distal renal tubular acidosis
- ☐ Renal papillary necrosis
- ☐ Diabetic nephropathy
- ☐ Analgesic nephropathy
- ☐ Renal osteodystrophy

GASTROENTEROLOGY REVISION INDEX

Numbers refer to question numbers.

Acid secretion 1
AIDS, gastrointestinal infections in 9
Anaemia, pernicious 4

Bilirubin 24

c-ret oncogene 25
Carcinoma, colorectal 7
Carcinoma, hepatocellular 12
Cholecystokinin 20
Chronic pancreatitis 14
Clostridium difficile 13, 33
Coeliac disease 11
Colorectal carcinoma 7

Delayed gastric emptying 32

Encephalopathy, hepatic 16, 18

Fat, dietary 30
Folic acid 15

Gastric emptying, delayed 32
Gastrin 1
Gastritis, chronic atrophic 4
Gastro-oesophageal reflux 26

Helicobacter pylori 10
Hepatic encephalopathy 16,18
Hepatitis, acute 21
Hepatitis C 17
Hepatocellular carcinoma 12
Hirschsprung's disease 25
Hypertension, portal 5

Intestinal pseudo-obstructions, chronic 8
Irritable bowel syndrome 22

Kaposi's sarcoma, gastrointestinal 9

Mesalazine compounds 31

Octreotide 6
Oesophageal varices, bleeding 5
Omeprazole 27
Overdose, paracetamol 3

Pancreatitis, chronic 14
Paracetamol 3
Parenteral nutrition 29
Pernicious anaemia 4
Portal hypertension 5
Primary biliary cirrhosis 2
Pseudomembranous colitis 13

Rectal ulcer 19

Shilling test 4
Solitary rectal ulcer syndrome 19
Systemic sclerosis 28

Total parenteral nutrition 29

Wilson's disease 23

Zollinger-Ellison syndrome 25

ENDOCRINOLOGY REVISION INDEX

Numbers refer to question numbers.

Acromegaly, 40
    active 39
Addison's disease 55, 59
ADH 41
Adrenal carcinoma 53
Adrenal hyperplasia, congenital 57
Anorexia nervosa 44
Antidiuretic hormone 41, 42
Atrial natriuretic peptide 54

Carcinoma, adrenal 53
Congenital adrenal hyperplasia 45, 57
Conn's syndrome 56
Craniopharyngioma 35
Cushing's syndrome 52, 53

DDAVP 66
de Quervain's post-viral thyroiditis 49
Di George syndrome 59
Diabetes insipidus 42

G-proteins 51
Galactorrhoea 43
Gastrinoma 66
Graves' disease 47
Growth hormone 37
    deficiency 64

Hirsutism 45
Hypercalcaemia 58
Hypercortisolism 52
Hyperparathyroidism 58
Hyperprolactinaemia 43
Hyperthyroidism 50

Hypoglycaemia 63
Hypokalaemia 56
Hypoparathyroidism, idiopathic 59
Hypopituitarism 38
Hypothyroidism, primary autoimmune 48

IGF-1 36
Insulin-like growth factor-1 36
Insulinomas 63

Kallman's syndrome 46
Klinefelter's syndrome 46

McCune Albright syndrome 51
Multiple endocrine neoplasia 62
Myxoedema 48

Osteoporosis 60

Paget's disease 61
Parathyroid hormone 58
Phaeochromocytoma 65
Pituitary fossa 34

Schmidt's syndrome 48

Thyroid stimulating hormone 47, 50
Thyrotoxicosis 49

Verner-Morrison syndrome 62

NEPHROLOGY REVISION INDEX

Numbers refer to question numbers.

Acute renal failure 67
Adult polycystic kidney disease 92
Albuminuria 97
Alport's syndrome 81
Altitude, effects of 77
ANCA 87
Anti-glomerular basement
    membrane disease 87
ATN 67, 68

Calculi, renal tract 98
CAPD 79
Carcinoma, renal 91
Cholesterol emboli 90
Chronic renal failure, drugs in 99
Clearance 75
Continuous ambulatory peritoneal
    dialysis 79
Cysts,
    hepatic 92
    pancreatic 92

Dialysis 80
Distal renal tubular acidosis 98
Drugs, and chronic renal failure
    99

End-stage renal failure 100

Genetically-transmitted diseases
    94
GFR 73, 74
Glomerular filtration rate 73, 74
Glomerulonephritis, rapidly
    progressive 87
Glomerulosclerosis 81
    chronic 84

    focal 84
Glomerular filtration 73
Goodpasture's syndrome 87

Haemolytic-uraemic syndrome 86
Hepatic cysts 92
Hepatorenal syndrome 69
Hyperparathyroidism 93
Hyperphosphataemia 93

IgA nephropathy 89
Interstitial nephritis 81
    acute allergic 70

Kidney disease, adult polycystic
    92
Kidney, normal 71

Loin pain-haematuria 89

Membranous glomerulonephritis
    88
Microalbuminuria, diabetic 97

Nephritis, interstitial 81
Nephrocalcinosis 98
Nephropathy 89
Nephrotic syndrome 90
Noonan's syndrome 94

Osteodystrophy, uraemic 93

Pancreatic cysts 92
Paraquat 67
Peripheral neuropathy 80
Polycystic kidney disease, adult
    92

Pregnancy, renal function in 74

Reflux, vesico-ureteric 95
Renal carcinoma 91
Renal failure 68, 82
    acute 67, 70
    chronic 83, 84
    end-stage 100
Renal function in pregnancy 74
Renal obstruction 85
Renal tract, calculi 98
    imaging 85
Renal tubular acidosis 98
Renin 78

SLE 82
Sodium, urinary excretion of 76

Tetracyclines 99
Thrombosis, renal vein 91
Tuberculosis 96
Type 1 renal tubular acidosis 98

Uraemia 80, 81
Uraemic osteodystrophy 93
Urinary tract
    infection 95
    tuberculosis of 96

Vesico-ureteric reflux 94, 95
von Hippel-Lindau syndrome 94

Water, renal excretion of 72
Wegener's granulomatosis 82